GRATITUDE JOURNAL
CONTENTS

POWER
THE POWER OF A GRATEFUL HEART

QUOTES
GRATITUDE QUOTES

PRAYER
GRATITUDE PRAYER

VERSES
GRATITUDE BIBLE VERSES

LIST
GRATITUDE LIST

IMAGES
GRATITUDE IMAGES

40 DAYS GRATITUDE JOURNAL

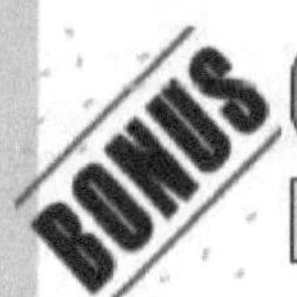

BONUS CHANGING YOUR THOUGHTS WILL CHANGE YOUR LIFE

POWERFUL TECHNIQUE TO ERASE PAINFUL MEMORIES

Writing

<> Find the right space to write
<> Close your eyes and reflect on your day
<> Ask yourself questions
<> Dive in and start writing
<> Time yourself
<> Re-read your entry and add additional thoughts

Prompts

What's something that you're looking forward to?
What's a simple pleasure that you're grateful for?
What's something that you are grateful to have today that you didn't have a year ago?
Write about a happy memory.
What's an accomplishment you're proud of?
What's a possession that makes your life easier?
What have you been given that you're grateful for?
What do you like about your job?
How are you able to help others?
What book(s) are you grateful for?
Write about a friend that you're grateful for.
What did you accomplish today?
What's a tradition that you're grateful for?
What mistake or failure are you grateful for?
What skill(s) do you have that you're grateful for?
What's something that you bought or received recently that you're grateful for?
Look around the room and write about everything you see that you're grateful for.
Write about 3 things you're grateful for today.

The Power of a Grateful Heart

We have so much to be grateful for in this life. Each and every day. But the reality is that many times constant life demands, struggles, and worries give more room to defeat than to a heart of thanks.

We have a choice, every day, to give God thanks. And with a heart of thanksgiving, we realize that no matter what we face, God doesn't just work to change our situations and help us through our problems.

He does more. Much, much more.

He changes our hearts. His power, through hearts of gratitude and focused minds on Him, releases the grip our struggles have over us.

We're strengthened by His peace, refueled by His joy.

God's word is filled with many reminders of how powerful and vital a thankful heart can be in this world.

Being grateful gets our eyes off ourselves, and helps us to focus back on God.

Being grateful reminds us that we're not in control. We serve a Mighty God who is.

Being grateful keeps us in a place of humility and dependency on Him as we recognize how much we need Him.

Being grateful helps us to recognize we have so much to be thankful for, even all of the little things, which often we may forget to thank Him for. But they really are the biggest, most important things in this life.

Being grateful takes our attention off of our problems and helps us instead to reflect on and to remember, the goodness of His many blessings.

Being grateful reminds us that God is the Giver of all good gifts. We were never intended to be fully self-sufficient in this life.

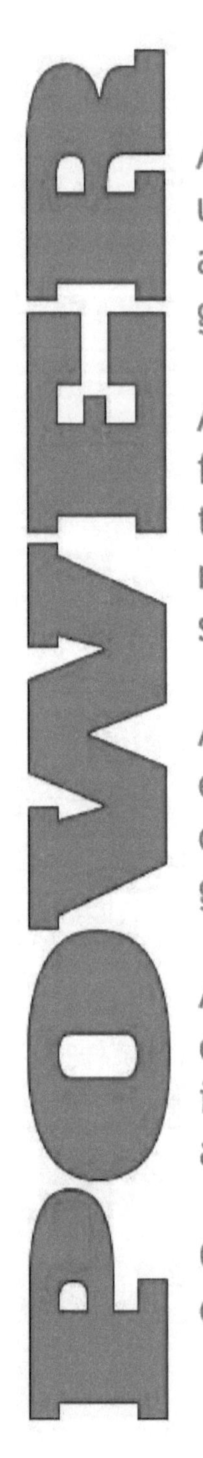

A grateful heart reminds us that ultimately God is our Provider, that all blessings and gifts are graciously given to us by His hand.

A heart of gratitude leaves no room for complaining, for it is impossible to be truly thankful and filled with negativity and ungratefulness at the same time.

A heart of gratitude makes the enemy flee. The forces of darkness can't stand to be around hearts that give thanks and honor to God.

A heart of gratitude opens up the door for continued blessings. It invites God's presence. Our spirits are refreshed and renewed in Him.

God loves to give good gifts to His children.

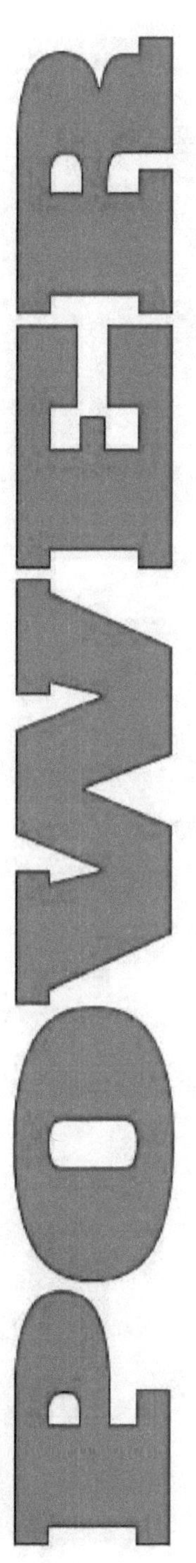

God delights in our thankfulness and pours out His Spirit and favor over those who give honor and show gratitude to Him.

In the midst of busyness and pressures, just to pause and give thanks, for all that God has done and continues to do in your live and in the lives of your loved ones.

POWER

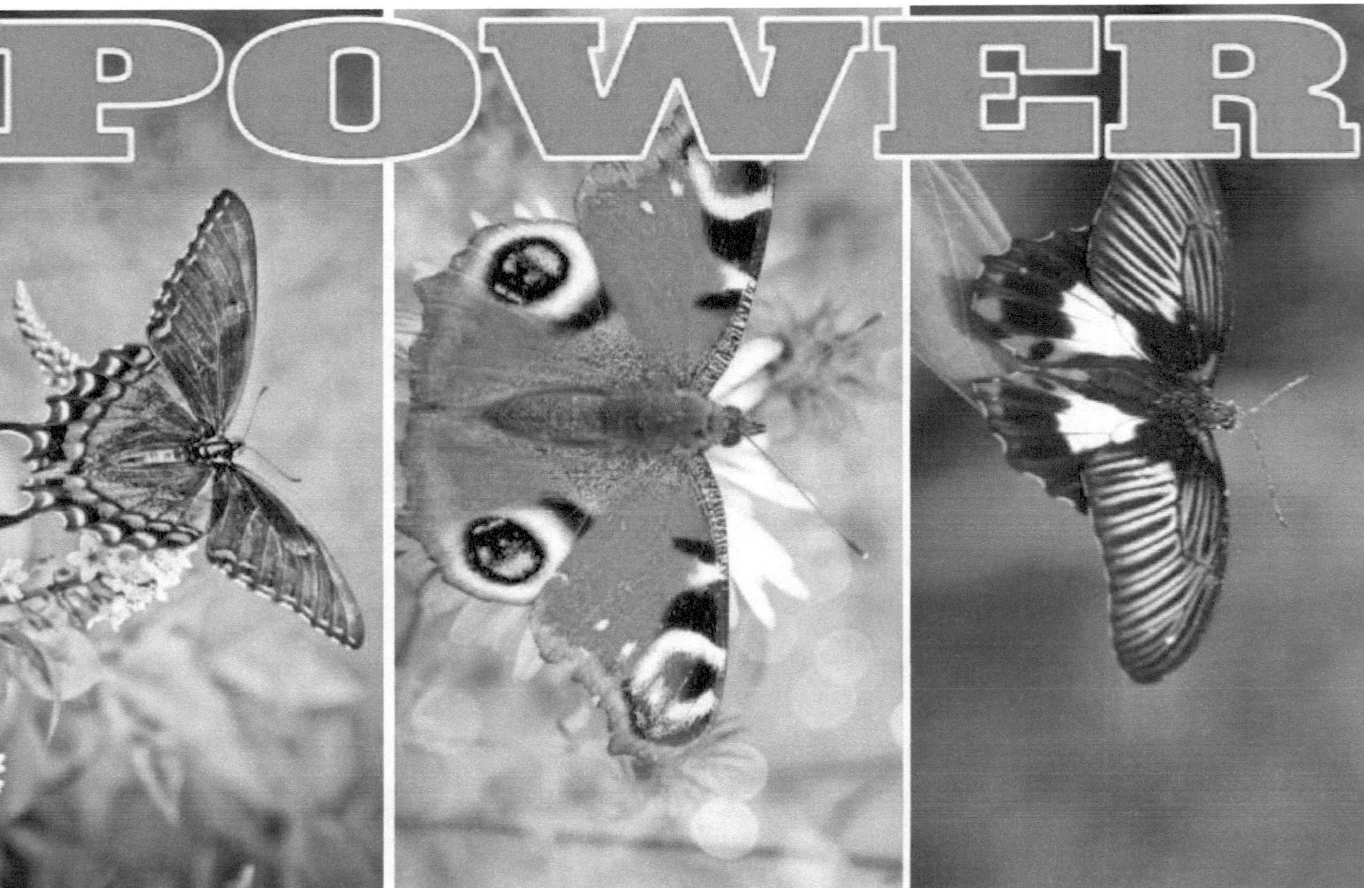

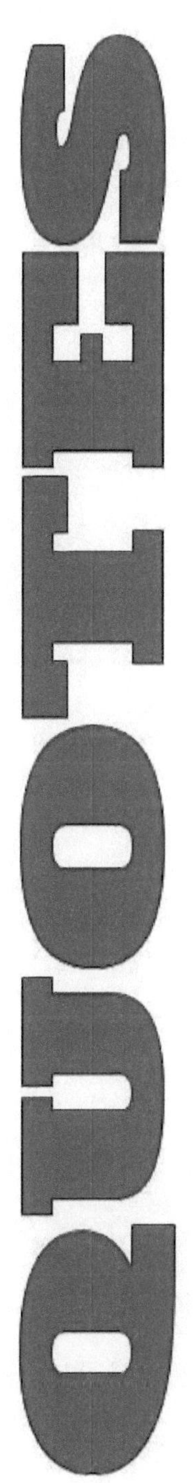

Gratitude Quotes

"Gratitude is not only the greatest of virtues but the parent of all others."
— Cicero

"I was complaining that I had no shoes till I met a man who had no feet."
— Confucius

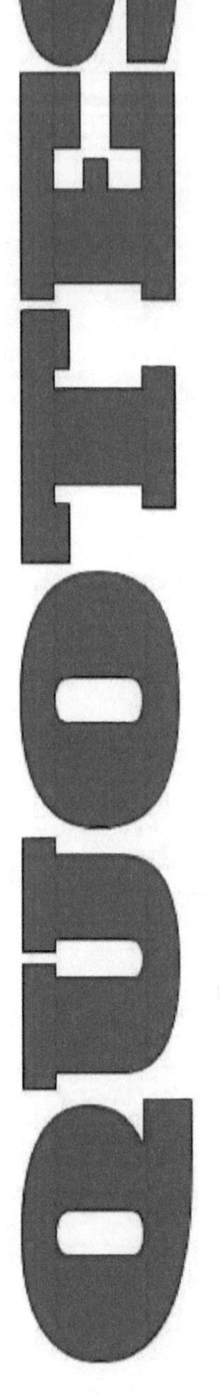

"Gratitude opens the door to the power, the wisdom, the creativity of the universe. You open the door through gratitude."
— Deepak Chopra

Appreciation is a wonderful thing: It makes what is excellent in others belong to us as well."
— Voltaire

"An attitude of gratitude brings great things."
— Yogi Bhajan

"It is not joy that makes us grateful, it is gratitude that makes us joyful."
— David Steindl-Rast

"Don't pray when it rains if you don't pray when the sun shines."
— Leroy Satchel Paige

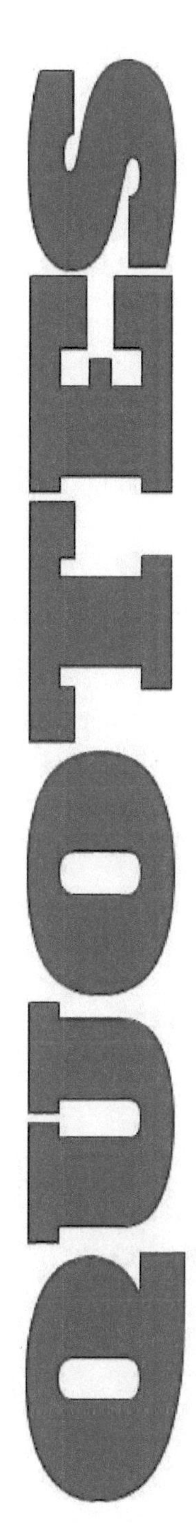

"It is only with gratitude that life becomes rich."
— Deitrich Bonheiffer

"We can choose to be grateful no matter what."
— Dieter F. Uchtdorf

"Entitlement is such a cancer, because it is void of gratitude."
— Adam Smith

"Gratitude changes everything."
— Anonymous

"Gratitude is riches. Complaint is poverty."
— Doris Day

"Gratitude is the sign of noble souls."
— Aesop

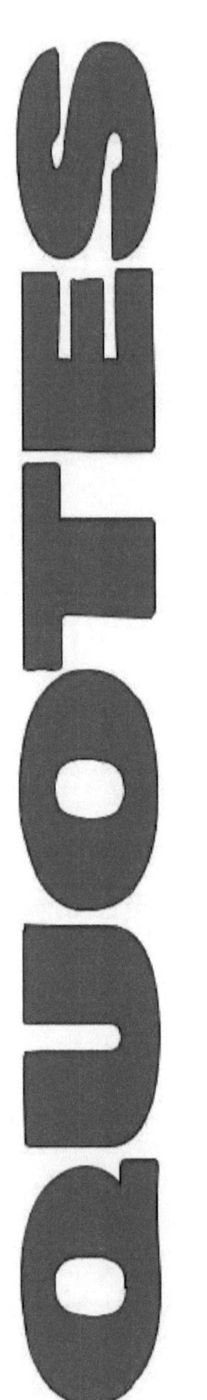

"Gratitude turns what we have into enough."
— Aesop

"Happiness is itself a kind of gratitude."
— Anonymous

"My day begins and ends with gratitude."
— Louise Hay

"The essence of all beautiful art is gratitude."
— Friedrich Nietzche

"The struggle ends when gratitude begins."
— Neale Donald Walsch

"Through the eyes of gratitude, everything is a miracle."
— Mary Davis

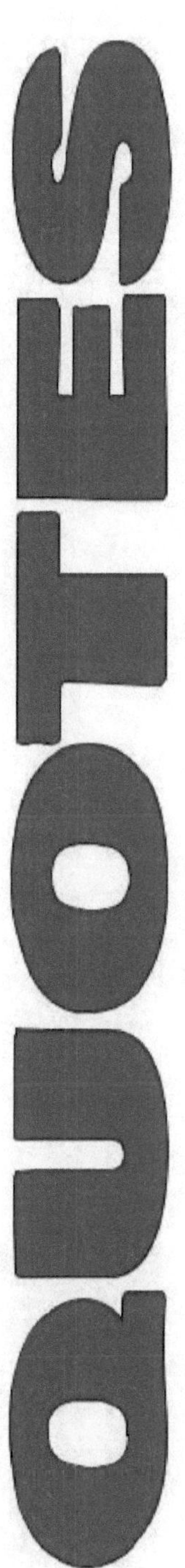

"Gratitude, like faith, is a muscle. The more you use it, the stronger it grows, and the more power you have to use it on your behalf. If you do not practice gratefulness, its benefaction will go unnoticed, and your capacity to draw on its gifts will be diminished. To be grateful is to find blessings in everything. This is the most powerful attitude to adopt, for there are blessings in everything."
— Alan Cohen

QUOTES

Gratitude Prayer

Thank you, Lord, for the blessings you have bestowed on my life.

You have provided me with more than I could ever have imagined. You have surrounded me with people who always look out for me.

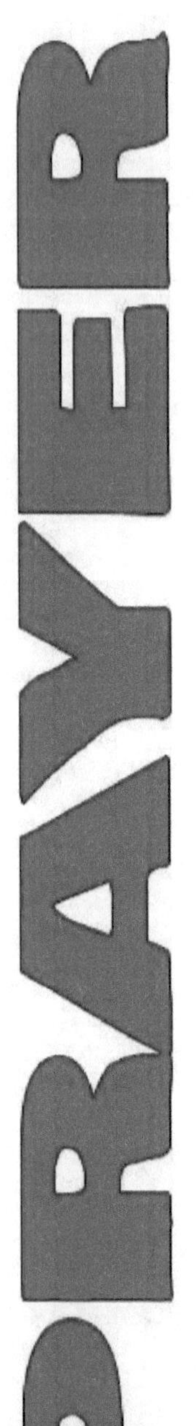

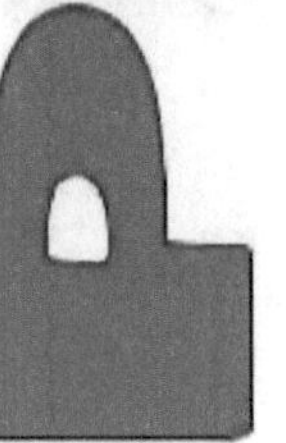

You have given me family and friends who bless me every day with kind words and actions. They lift me up in ways that keep my eyes focused on you and make my spirit soar.

Also, thank you, Lord, for keeping me safe. You protect me from those things that seem to haunt others. You help me make better choices, and you have provided me with advisors that help me with the difficult decisions.

You speak to me in so many ways so that I always know you are here.

And Lord, I am so grateful for keeping those around me safe and loved.

I hope that you provide me with the ability and sense to show them every day how much they matter.

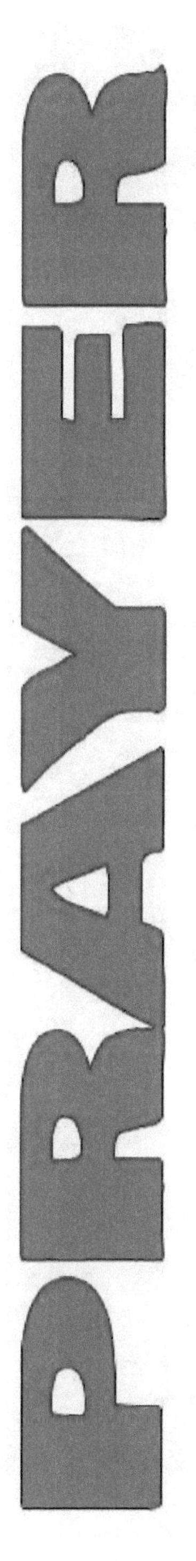

I hope that you give me the ability to give to them the same kindness they have provided to me.

I am just so grateful for all of your blessings in my life, Lord.

I pray that you remind me of just how lucky I am, and that you never allow me to forget to show my gratitude in prayer and returned kind acts.

Thank you,

Amen

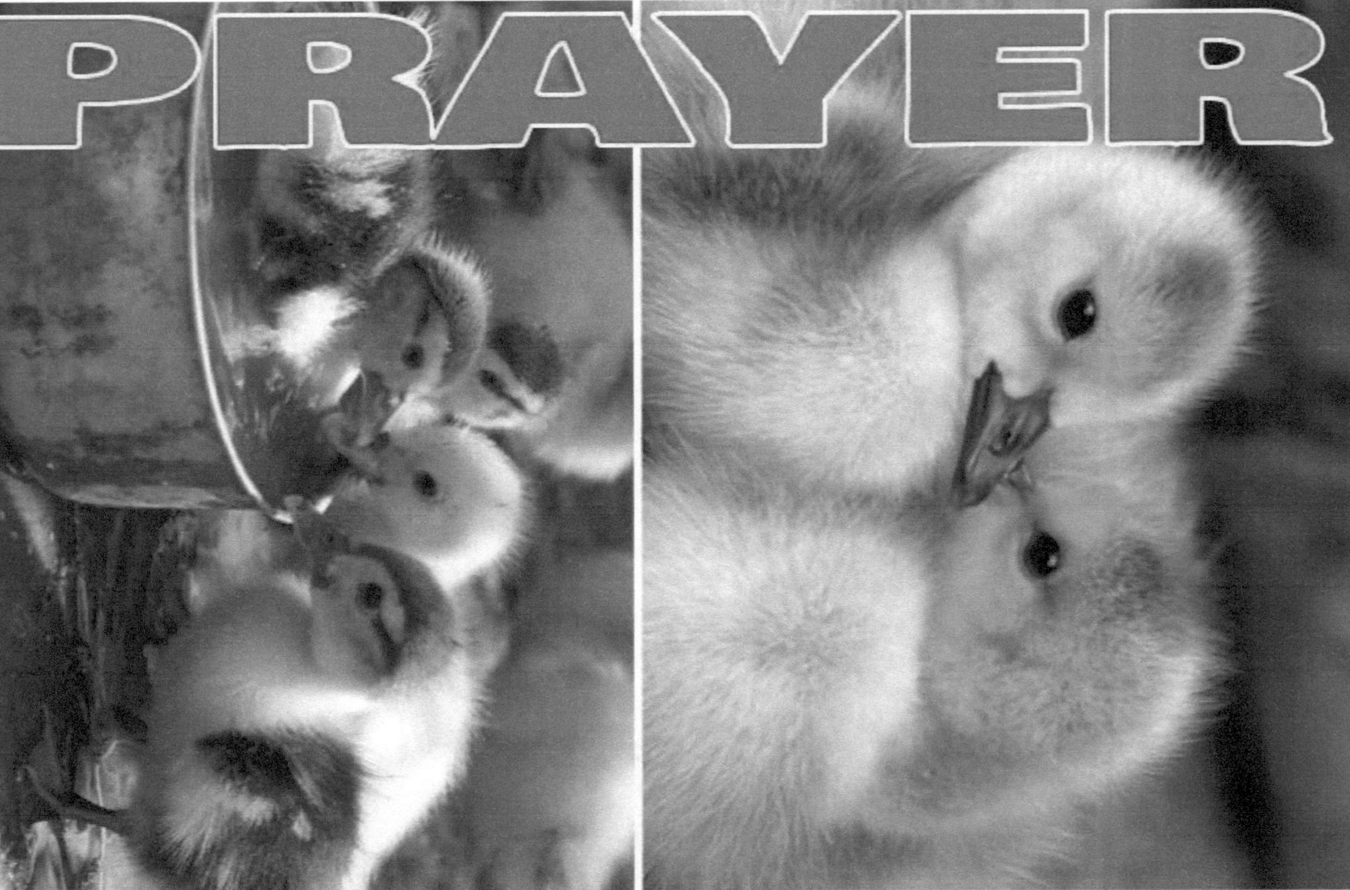
PRAYER

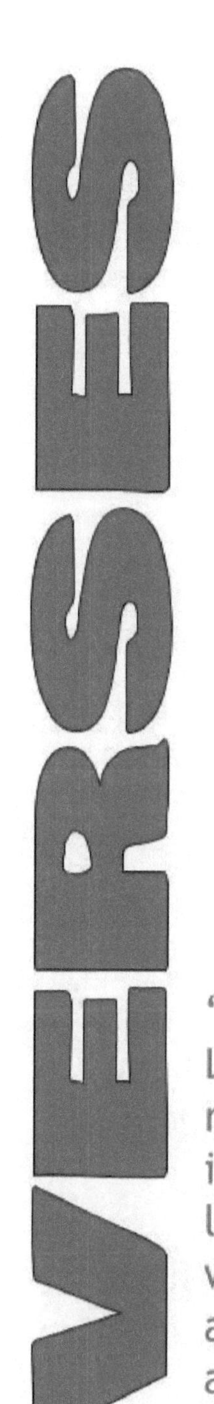

Gratitude Bible Verses

"O Come, let us sing for joy to the Lord; Let us shout joyfully to the rock of our salvation. Let us come into his presence with thanksgiving; let us make a joyful noise to him with songs of praise! For the Lord is a great God, and a great King above all gods." Ps. 95:1-3

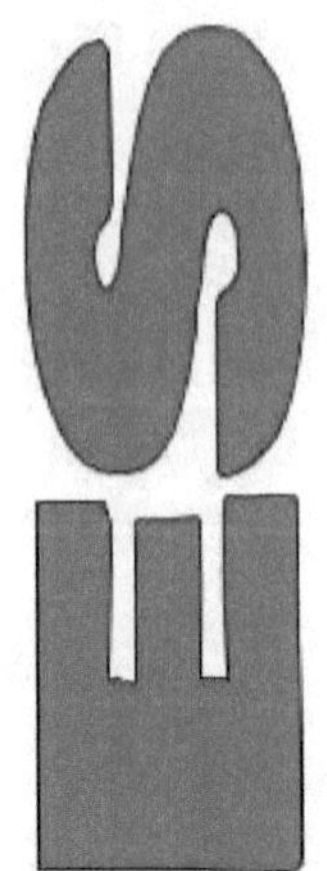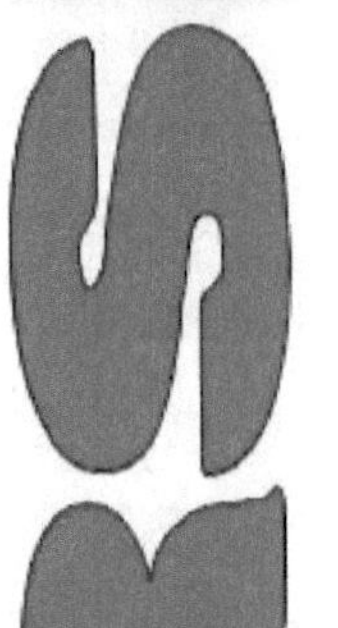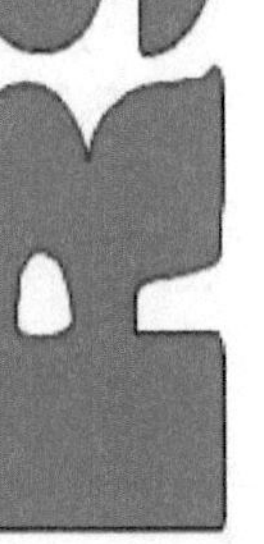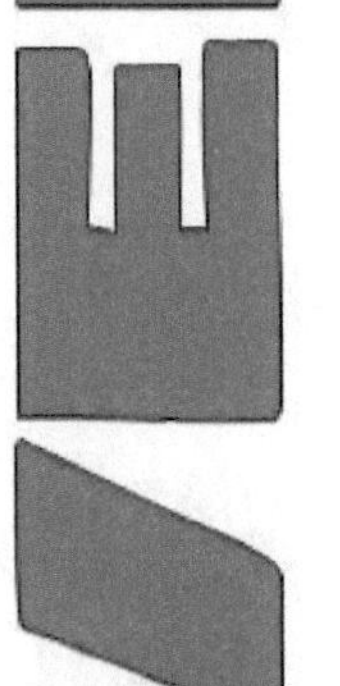

"Enter his gates with thanksgiving, and his courts with praise! Give thanks to him; bless his name! For the Lord is good; his steadfast love endures forever, and his faithfulness to all generations." Ps. 100:4-5

"I will give thanks to you, LORD, with all my heart; I will tell of all your wonderful deeds." Ps. 9:1

"I will give to the Lord the thanks due to his righteousness, and I will sing praise to the name of the Lord, the Most High." Ps. 7:17

"And let the peace of Christ rule in your hearts, to which indeed you were called in one body; and be thankful." Col. 3:15

"Give thanks to the Lord for he is good, his love endures forever." Ps. 118:29

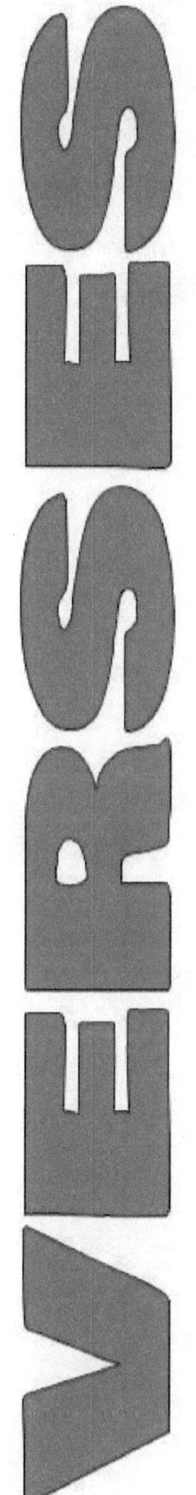

"Let your roots grow down into him, and let your lives be built on him. Then your faith will grow strong in the truth you were taught, and you will overflow with thankfulness." Col. 2:7

"Every good gift and every perfect gift is from above, coming down from the Father of lights with whom there is no variation or shadow due to change." James 1:17

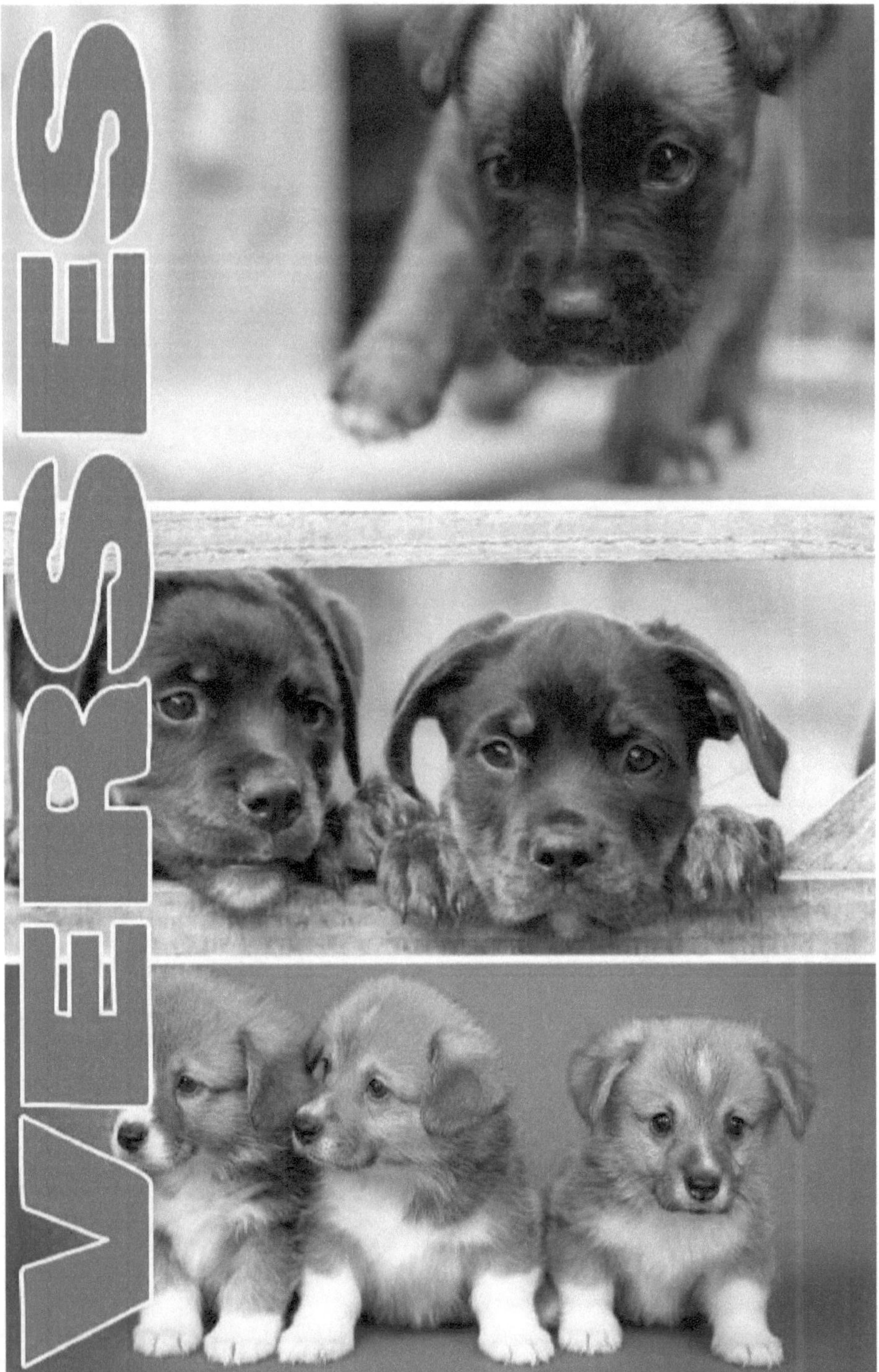

VERSES

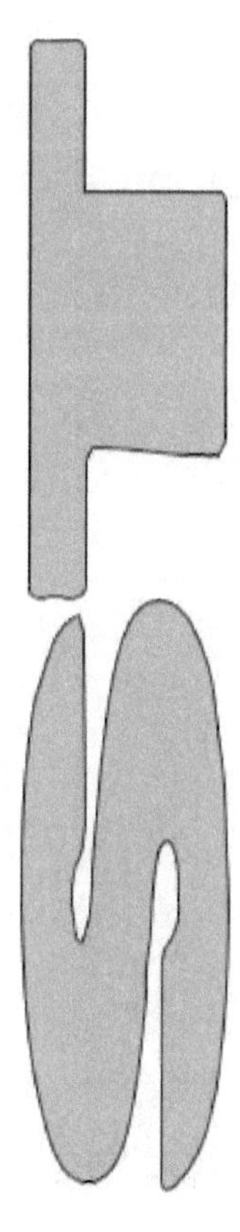

Gratitude List

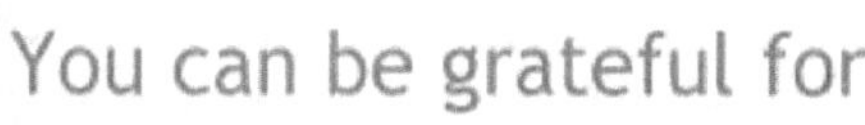

You can be grateful for

- ❏ God, Jesus and the Holy Spirit that are in you, an unlimited resource to achieve everything
- ❏ Your Parents – for giving birth to you. Because if there is no them, there will not be you

- ❏ Your Family – for being your closest kin in the world
- ❏ Your Friends – for being your companions in life
- ❏ Your Sense of Sight – for letting you see the colors of life
- ❏ Your Sense of Hearing – for letting you hear trickle of rain, the voices of your loved ones, and the harmonious music
- ❏ Your Sense of Touch – for letting you feel the texture of your clothes, the breeze of the wind, the hands of your loved ones
- ❏ Your Sense of Smell – for letting you smell scented candles, perfumes, and beautiful flowers in your garden
- ❏ Your Sense of Taste – for letting you savor the sweetness of fruits, the saltiness of seawater, the sourness of pickles, and the spiciness of chili

- Your Speech - for giving you the outlet to express yourself
- Your Heart - for pumping blood to all the parts of your body every second since you were born and for the ability to feel
- Your Lungs - for letting you breathe so you can live
- Your Immune System - for fighting viruses that enter your body and for keeping you in the pink of your health so you can do the things you love
- Your Hands - so you can type on your computer, flip the pages of books, and hold the hands of your loved ones
- Your Legs - for letting you walk, run, swim, play the sports you love, and curl up in the comfort of your seat
- Your Mind - for the ability to think, to store memories, and to create new solutions

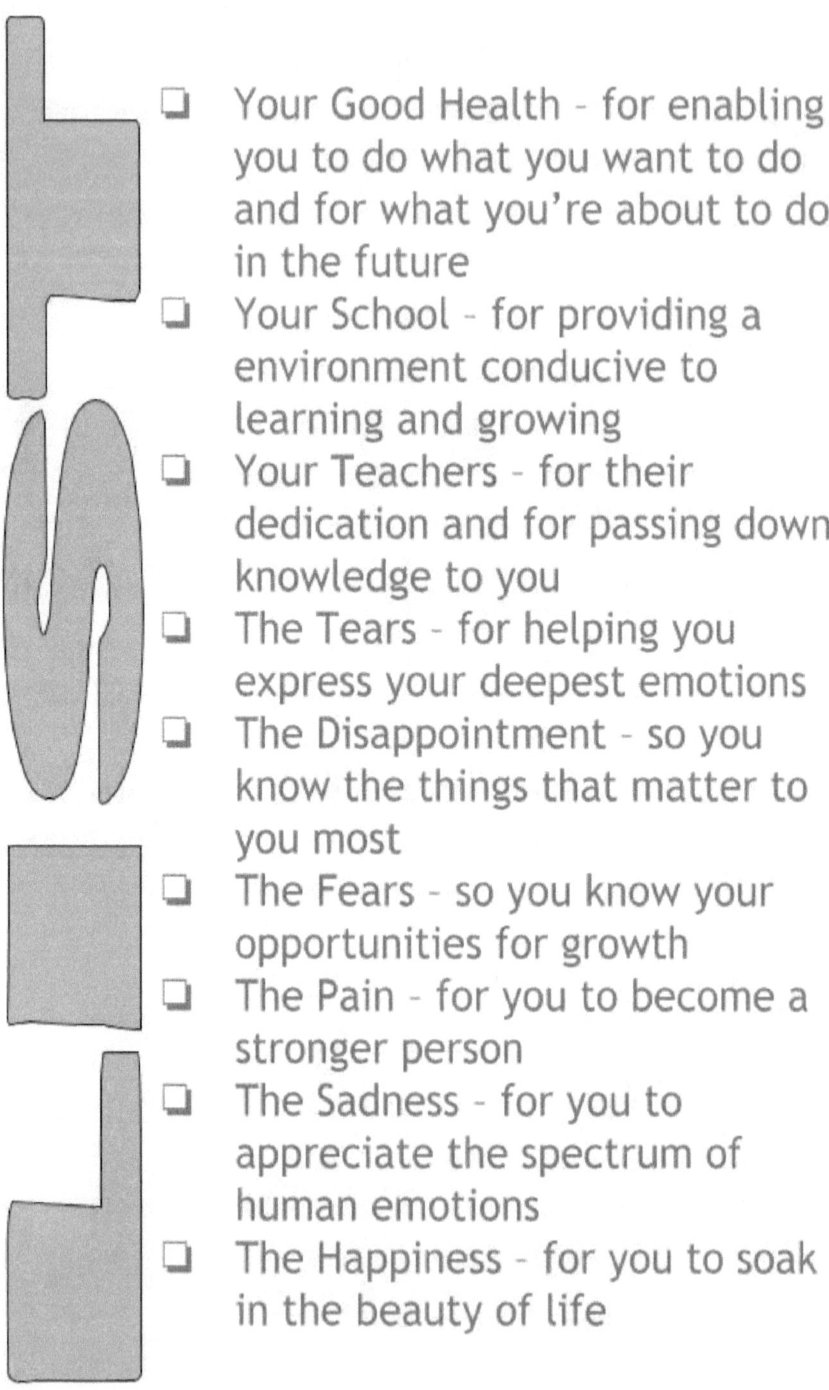

- ❏ Your Good Health – for enabling you to do what you want to do and for what you're about to do in the future
- ❏ Your School – for providing a environment conducive to learning and growing
- ❏ Your Teachers – for their dedication and for passing down knowledge to you
- ❏ The Tears – for helping you express your deepest emotions
- ❏ The Disappointment – so you know the things that matter to you most
- ❏ The Fears – so you know your opportunities for growth
- ❏ The Pain – for you to become a stronger person
- ❏ The Sadness – for you to appreciate the spectrum of human emotions
- ❏ The Happiness – for you to soak in the beauty of life

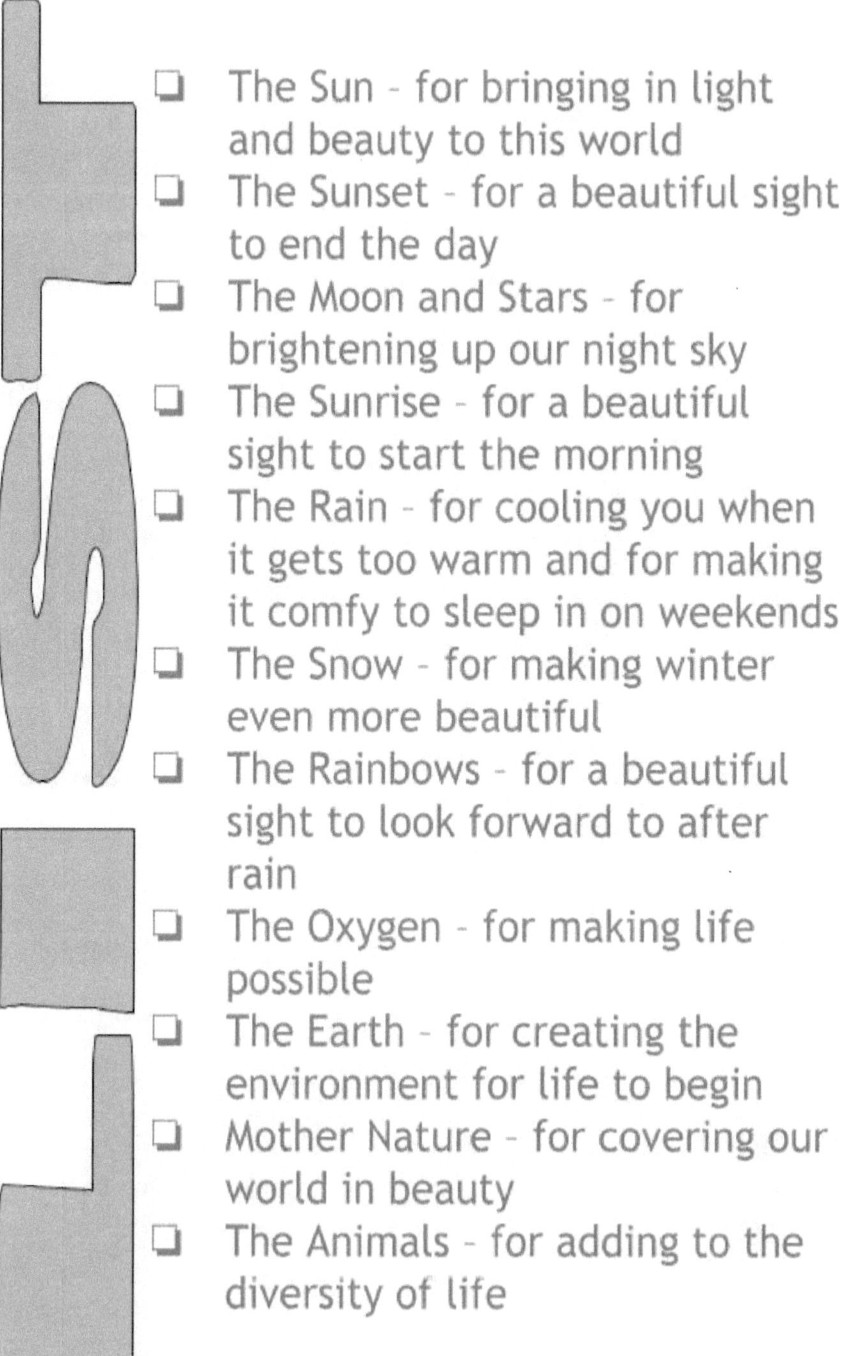

- ❏ The Sun – for bringing in light and beauty to this world
- ❏ The Sunset – for a beautiful sight to end the day
- ❏ The Moon and Stars – for brightening up our night sky
- ❏ The Sunrise – for a beautiful sight to start the morning
- ❏ The Rain – for cooling you when it gets too warm and for making it comfy to sleep in on weekends
- ❏ The Snow – for making winter even more beautiful
- ❏ The Rainbows – for a beautiful sight to look forward to after rain
- ❏ The Oxygen – for making life possible
- ❏ The Earth – for creating the environment for life to begin
- ❏ Mother Nature – for covering our world in beauty
- ❏ The Animals – for adding to the diversity of life

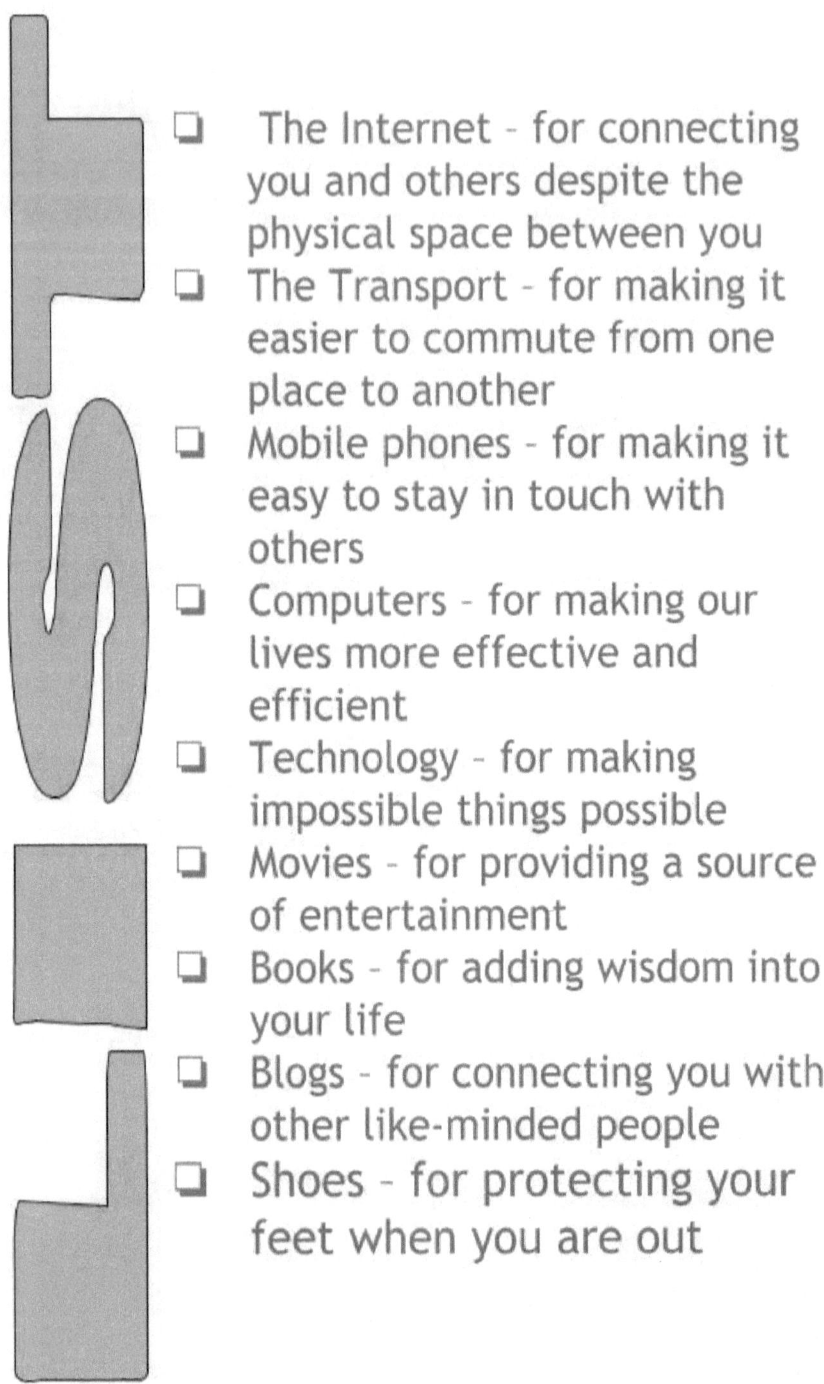

- The Internet – for connecting you and others despite the physical space between you
- The Transport – for making it easier to commute from one place to another
- Mobile phones – for making it easy to stay in touch with others
- Computers – for making our lives more effective and efficient
- Technology – for making impossible things possible
- Movies – for providing a source of entertainment
- Books – for adding wisdom into your life
- Blogs – for connecting you with other like-minded people
- Shoes – for protecting your feet when you are out

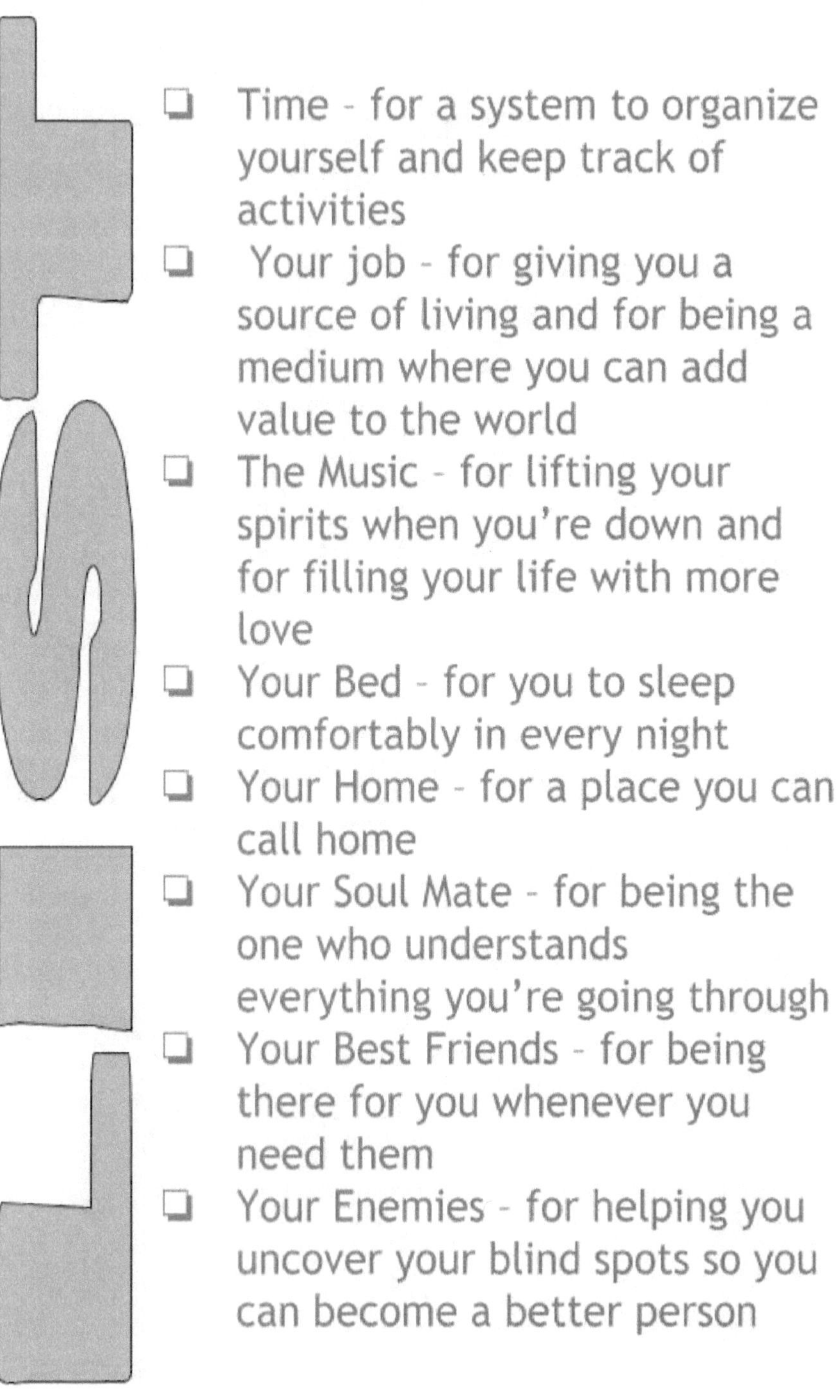

- ❏ Time – for a system to organize yourself and keep track of activities
- ❏ Your job – for giving you a source of living and for being a medium where you can add value to the world
- ❏ The Music – for lifting your spirits when you're down and for filling your life with more love
- ❏ Your Bed – for you to sleep comfortably in every night
- ❏ Your Home – for a place you can call home
- ❏ Your Soul Mate – for being the one who understands everything you're going through
- ❏ Your Best Friends – for being there for you whenever you need them
- ❏ Your Enemies – for helping you uncover your blind spots so you can become a better person

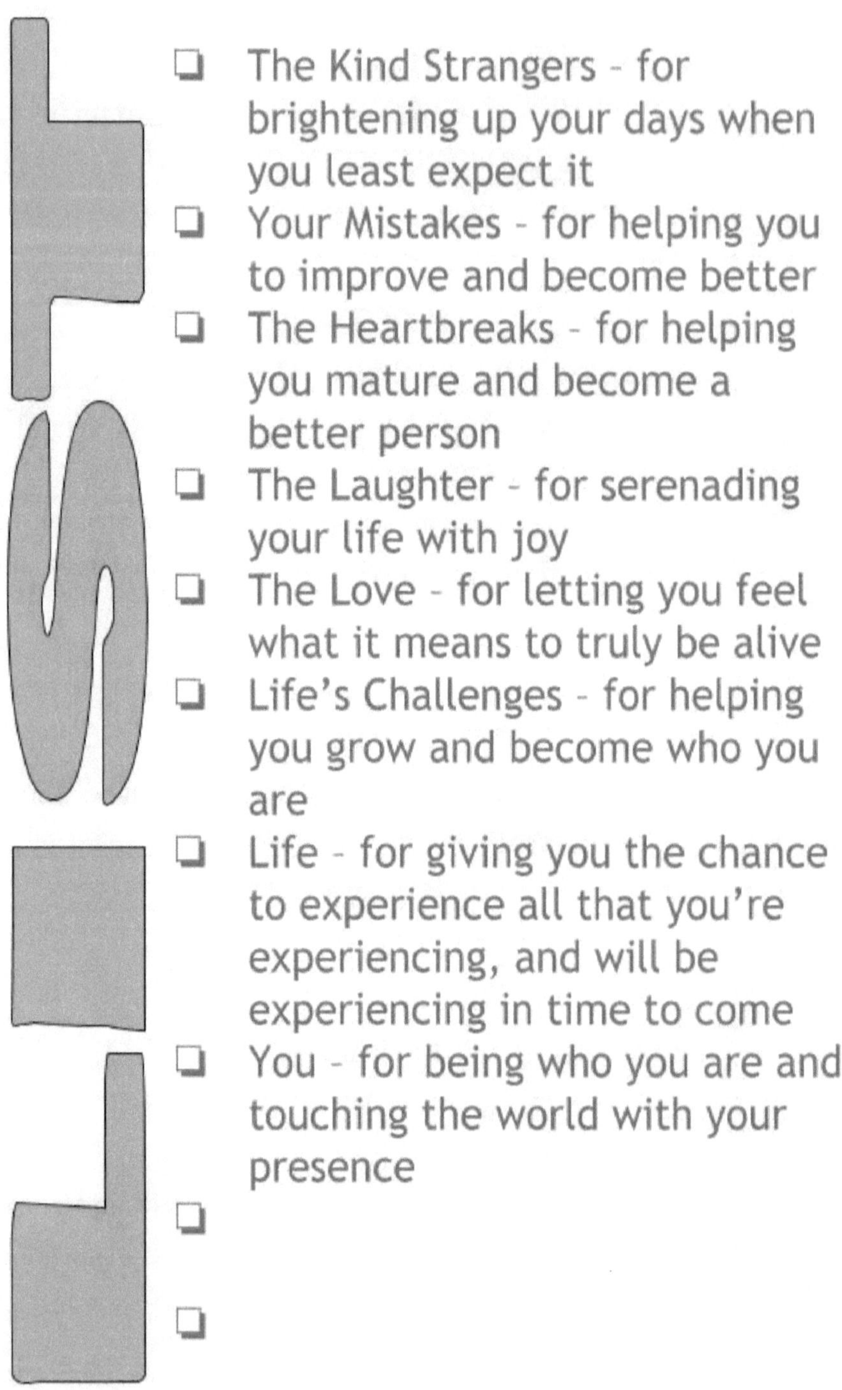

- ❏ The Kind Strangers – for brightening up your days when you least expect it
- ❏ Your Mistakes – for helping you to improve and become better
- ❏ The Heartbreaks – for helping you mature and become a better person
- ❏ The Laughter – for serenading your life with joy
- ❏ The Love – for letting you feel what it means to truly be alive
- ❏ Life's Challenges – for helping you grow and become who you are
- ❏ Life – for giving you the chance to experience all that you're experiencing, and will be experiencing in time to come
- ❏ You – for being who you are and touching the world with your presence
- ❏
- ❏

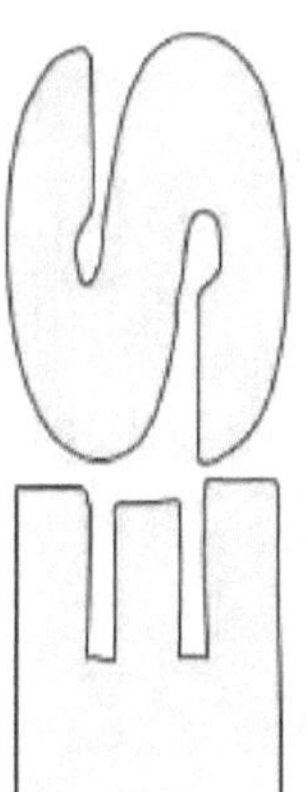

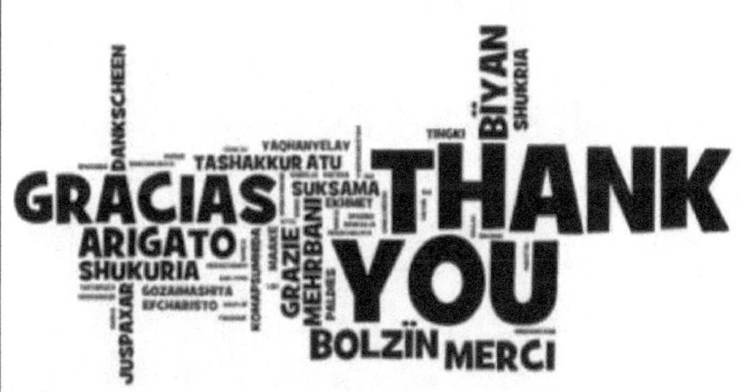
DANKSCHEEN
YAQHANYELAV
TASHAKKUR ATU
GRACIAS
ARIGATO
SHUKURIA
JUSPAXAR
GOZAMASHYA
EFCHARISTO
GRAZIE
MEHRBANI
SUKSAMA
EKOMET
TINGKI
BÏYAN
SHUKRIA
THANK
YOU
BOLZÏN
MERCI

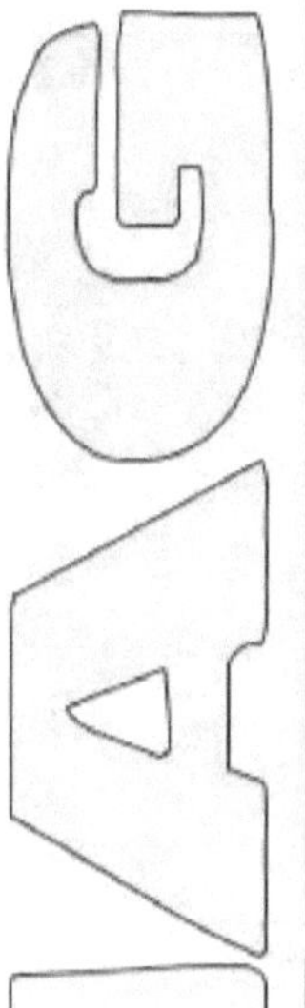

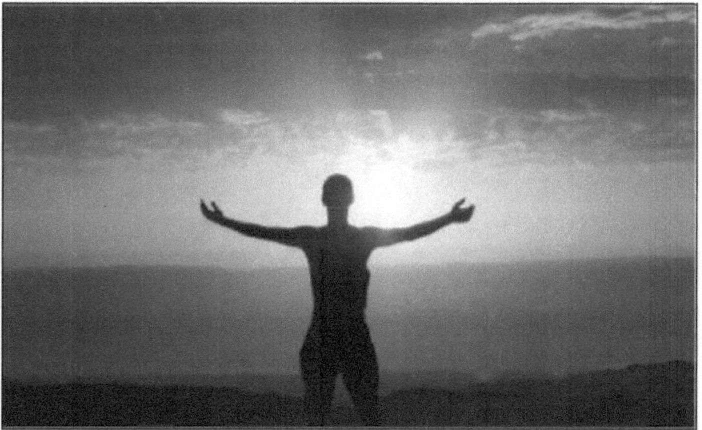

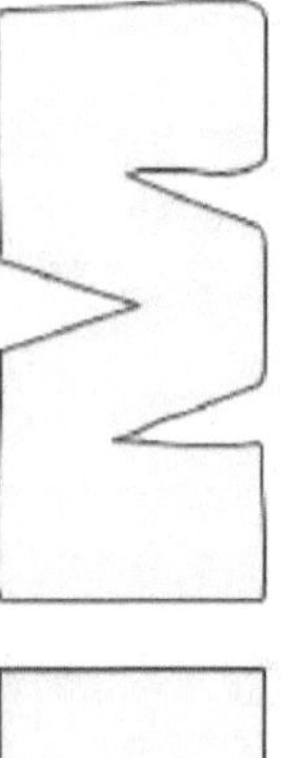

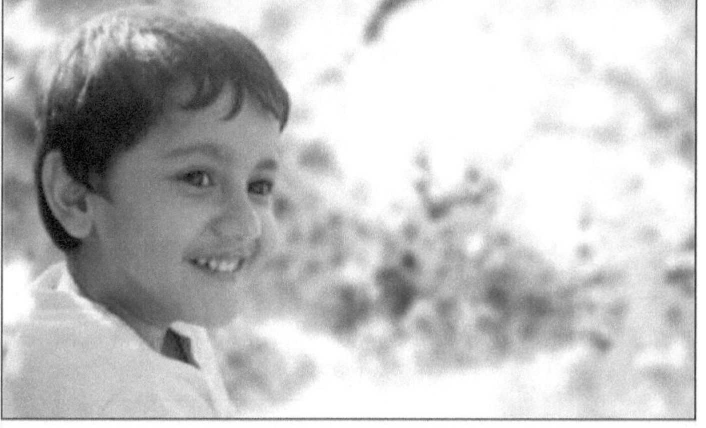

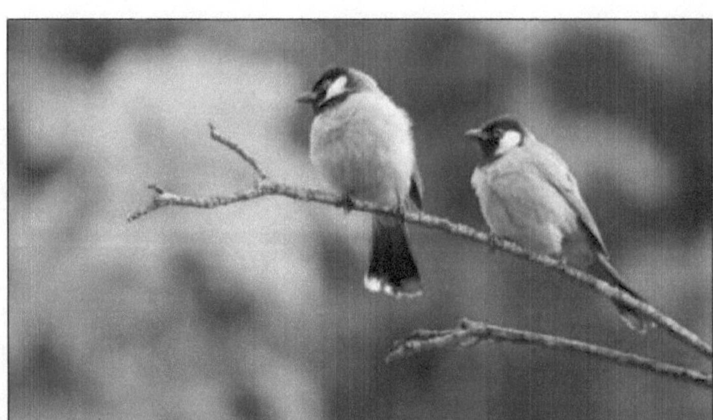

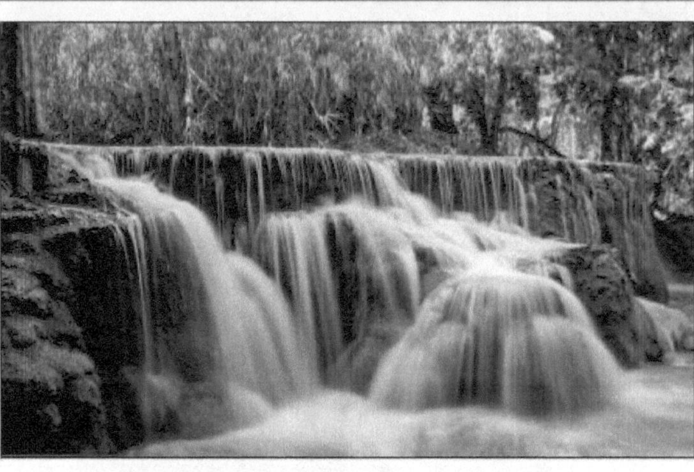

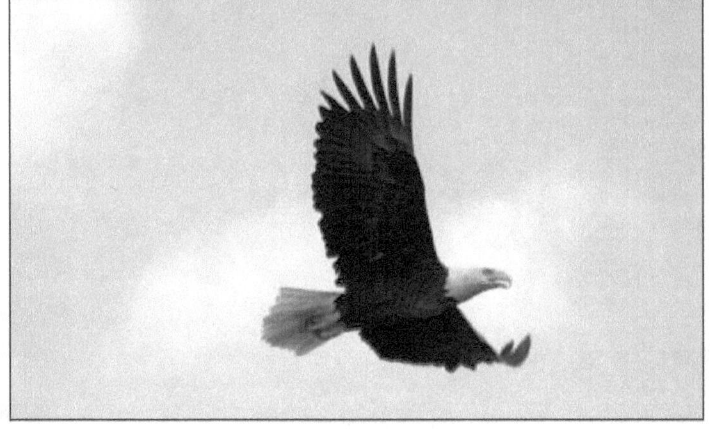

IMAGES

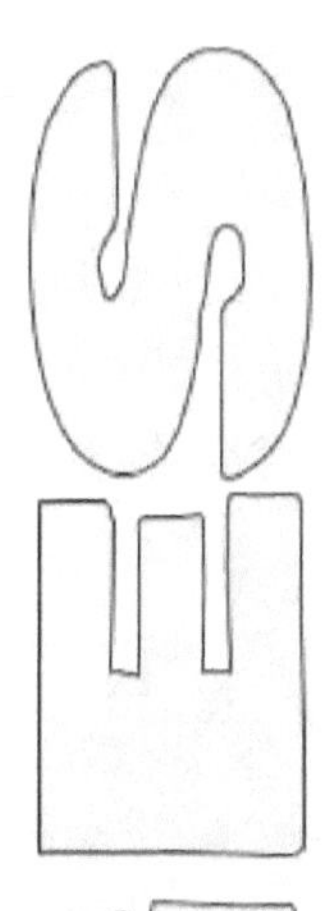

What do you want to do
that will improve the live
of other people?

...

What kind of legacy do
you want to leave?

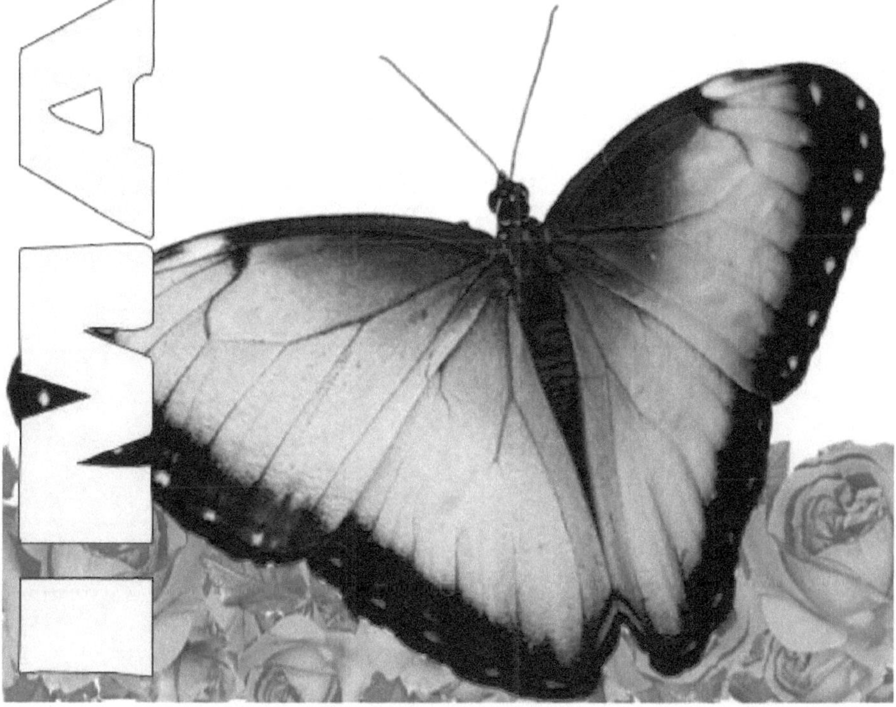

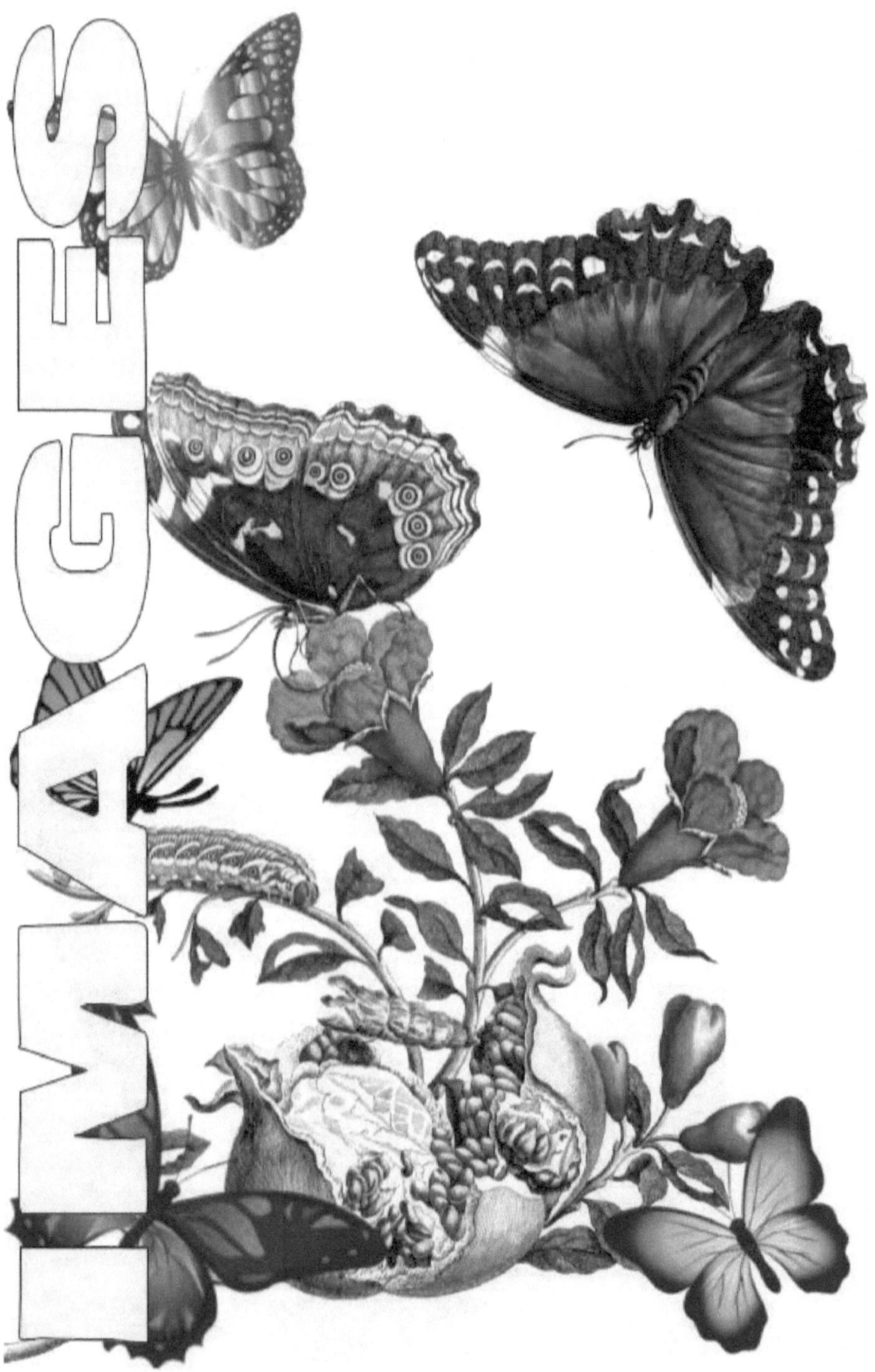

40 DAYS GRATITUDE JOURNAL

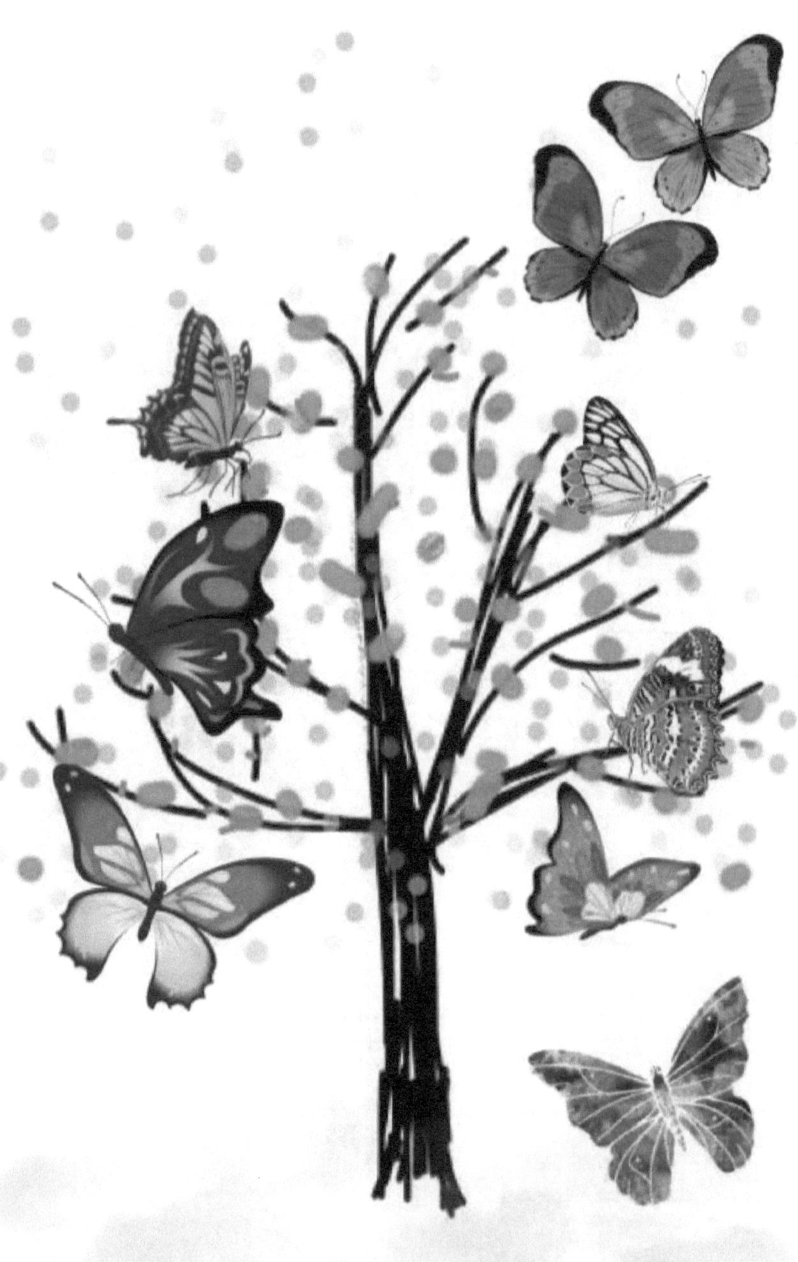

Changing Your Thoughts Will Change Your Life

If you are not happy with your destiny then you really must change your character.

But before you can change your character, you really must change your habits.

But before you can change your habits, you really must change your actions.

But before you can change your actions, you really must change your thoughts.

The key of your destiny (good or bad) lays on your own thoughts. Whatever you are today is the result of the thoughts you had during the last five years. Change your thoughts and your destiny will change.

Believe you will succeed and YOU
WILL, after all, deep in your core, you
are born to succeed.

Work on visualization, think of ways to
turn visualization into action, list the
reasons you will get what you want.

Stop being your own worst critic.

Believe in yourself.

On the next page you will learn a
powerful technique to erase painful
memories once and for all.

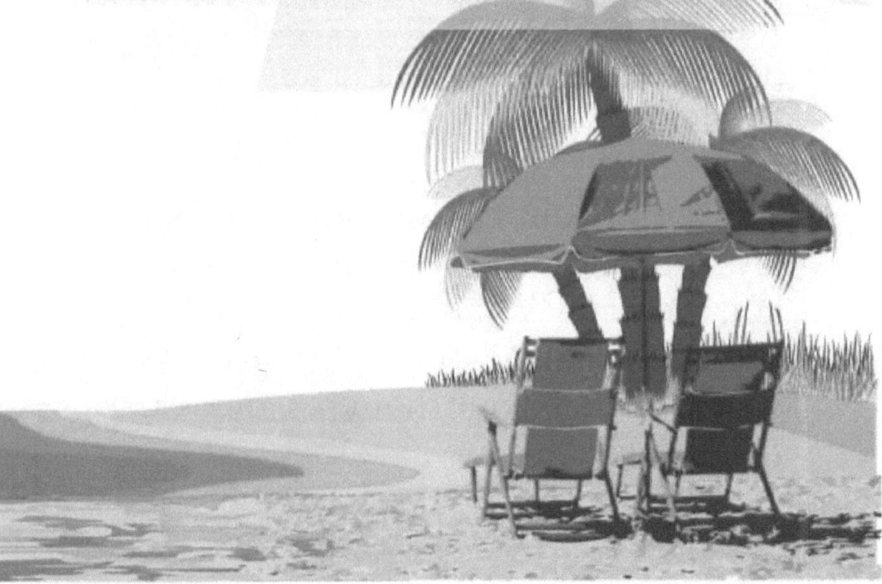

Powerful Technique to Erase Painful Memories

Step One
The first very important step is for you to **decide that you are done with that painful memory**. The rest of this exercise won't work if step one is not done properly. It is like a boxer preparing himself to go into the ring for this big fight. Next, find a peaceful spot and proceed with step two.

Step Two
Bring that painful memory for the last time, put a lot of colors everywhere, in their faces, in their clothing, overall, make it feel like a little boy or girl birthday party with happy music and everybody having a great time, and I mean _everybody_; remove the original voices and replace it with laughs and jokes; include your favorite toys when you were a child, your favorite spots for vacation, your favorite food or drink.

Step Three

Run this movie-memory backward full speed with circus music on the back, over and over and be sure to have fun with the images and the music.

Step Four

Visualize your new life surrounded by those that love and appreciate who you are, living in peace and with the job you like, the house you always wanted, the family you always wanted, the car, the plane, the bank account. Have a deep breath and sent this new energy out and believe that your are placing your order for your new life.

Boost this Technique

On the step one, you can write down that bad memory, find a place that brings you good memories and proceed to burn the paper with the bad memory while declaring that it is now out of your mind and your spirit is clean as the spirit of a new born baby.